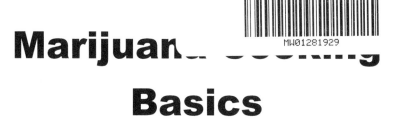

Marijuana Cooking Basics

Easy Sweet and Savory Weed Recipes

Cannabis Cookbook

George Green

ISBN: 9781792195389

Printed in the United States

Contents

Introduction

Cannabis is probably the most controversial plant we know about. Despite its plethora of medical applications, the plant is still most notorious for its recreational uses. However, well-known research organizations and nutritional experts across the world are working to better understand how cannabis impacts our bodies. Many people don't realize that cannabis extract and infusion-based products deliver many health benefits and prevent many diseases and disorders.

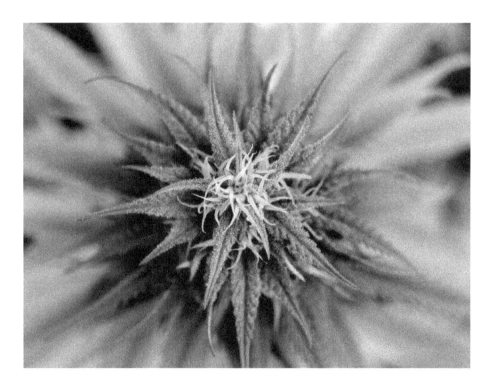

Welcome to the World of Cannabis

The cannabis plant contains many cannabinoid compounds, but the two most important ones are cannabidiol (CBD) and tetrahydrocannabinol (THC).

CBD is non-psychoactive, meaning that it does not deliver that "high" effect, but scientific experiments and studies have confirmed that it has a wide variety of medical uses. CBD helps to regulate the body's state of balance or "homeostasis". In short, it positively affects appetite, sleep, immune response, mood, and hormone regulation.

THC, on the other hand, does deliver that "high" effect. THC attaches to the cannabinoid receptors in the brain to cause psychological effects. It also influences certain areas of the brain that are responsible for pleasure, memory, and movement.

Taken together, THC and CBD work synergistically to optimize each other's curative properties. CBD activates the anti-cancer and analgesic properties of THC while reducing its psychoactivity. CBD can also ease rapid heartbeat, anxiety, and other adverse side effects caused by taking THC in large dosages.

Some pharmaceutical companies have successfully created cannabis-based drugs to treat certain health conditions and disorders. These drugs contain more CBD or THC according to their purpose. Cannabis is also being sold commercially in various forms such as tinctures, capsules, sprays, and topical creams.

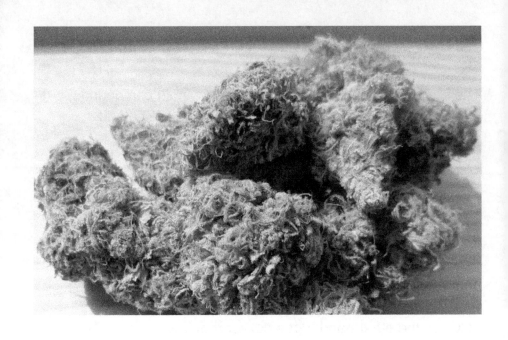

Cannabis: Medicinal Properties

Much research and many scientific studies, including a review published by the *British Journal of Pharmacology* in 2013, have discussed the possible medicinal properties of CBD. Most of these studies have been conducted on animals; only a few of them included human subjects.

The studies concluded that the use of cannabis may deliver the following medicinal effects:

Anti-inflammatory
Cannabis minimizes inflammation to prevent inflammatory disorders, including glaucoma. According to a review published by the National Eye Institute based in Bethesda, Maryland, cannabis aids in minimizing the pressure within the eyeball and thus helps control the symptoms of glaucoma, an eye condition marked by increased pressure within the eyeball, which leads to gradual loss of vision. Cannabis may decrease the pressure in the eye and prevent or delay vision loss.

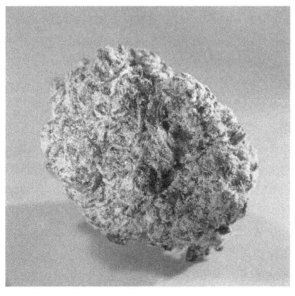

Respiratory Effects

A study published in the *Journal of the American Medical Association* in 2012 suggested that smoking cannabis does not hamper the function of the lungs. In fact, smoking cannabis may improve lung capacity.

Antipsychotic and Antidepressant

Cannabis fights various psychosis disorders, as well as the symptoms of depression and anxiety.

There has been much scientific research analyzing the effects of medical cannabis in controlling the symptoms of mental disorders such as anxiety, major depression, bipolar disorder, mania, panic disorder, schizophrenia, and other forms of psychosis.

A study conducted in 2006 by the *Molecular Pharmaceutics Journal* stated that cannabis can be effective in controlling the progression of Alzheimer's disease.

Anticonvulsant

In the mid-19th century, the *United States Pharmacopeia* described cannabis tincture as a valid treatment for pediatric epilepsy. Later studies indicated that the anticonvulsant properties of the cannabis plant may help minimize the frequency and intensity of temporal and parietal lobe seizures.

Antidiabetic

Studies have also found that cannabis positively affects fasting insulin and insulin resistance. Additional benefits listed by the American Alliance for Medical Cannabis (2005) include suggestions that it is a vasodilator and an antispasmodic agent, and that it relieves the symptoms of Restless Leg Syndrome (RLS) and neuropathic pain.

Antiemetic and Antioxidant

Cannabis protects against cell damage and oxidation, thereby preventing neurodegenerative diseases.

Cannabis consumption may help in relieving or controlling nausea and vomiting.

Anticancer/Anti-tumoral

Research from the California Pacific Medical Center appearing in the *Molecular Cancer Therapeutics* journal in 2007 reported that CBD may be effective in preventing the spread of cancer by shutting down a gene known as Id-This gene activates cancer cells and prompts them to spread throughout the body.

Multiple Sclerosis

Multiple sclerosis leads to many painful symptoms. Medical cannabis can be an effective option to minimize pain and muscle spasms.

Pain Relief

One of the most common uses of medical cannabis is for pain relief. THC may relieve pain by stimulating the pathways within the central nervous system that block the pain signals from reaching the brain.

Asthma

CBD may deliver potent immunosuppressive and anti-inflammatory effects that are extremely helpful in controlling the symptoms of asthma. THC may also help in calming asthma attacks.

Creative Cooking with Cannabis

Whether you are an experienced smoker, a recreational user, or just a cannabis enthusiast, there are many creative ways to give your taste buds a hint of cannabis.

Cannabis recipes offer a little medicated flavor and contain only a slight hint of cannabis. It takes 1–2 hours to feel the effects of ingested cannabis as THC enters the blood through the digestive system.

Cooking with Already Been Vaped (ABV) Cannabis

AVB (Already Vaped Bud), also popularly known as Already Been Vaped (ABV), is the plant matter that remains after cannabis is vaporized. Vaporizing is a different way of inhaling cannabis, similar to smoking. The two most common methods of preparing ABV are:

1) Manual Hot Water Technique
This involves submerging cannabis completely in a pot of hot water. Let the cannabis rest in the hot water for 30–45 minutes. Discard the water and preserve the cannabis. Heat more water in a separate pot and then add it to the cannabis pot. Again let it rest for 30–45 minutes. Repeat until the discarded water does not smell like cannabis. Dry out the cannabis at room temperature or in sunlight.

2) Cannabis Vaporizing Machine
This involves heating cannabis at 300–400°F using a cannabis vaporizing machine. When heated at these temperatures, cannabis releases the psychoactive compound THC. Vaporizing

is increasing in popularity as the technique prevents the inhalation of unwanted gases and tars that are released when smoking cannabis. These machines are different than water pipes.

Vaped cannabis is dark brown in color and has a subtle, distinct aroma in comparison to fresh cannabis buds. Many people simply discard ABV because they believe that they have already extracted all its essence and mood-enhancing benefits. However, you can still get more out of your ABV.

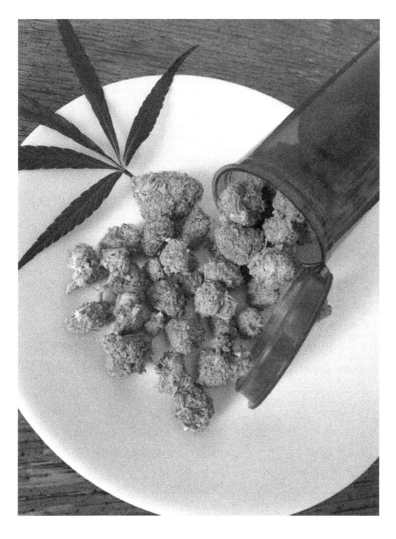

Decarboxylation (explained in the next section) is the chemical process that happens when cannabis gives up a carbon molecule, usually through heating. Until this happens, the plant has very little effect on people. As ABV has already been de-carbed, one can use it for several different purposes:

1) Smoking
You can smoke cannabis that has already been vaped, although not a lot of cannabis users do this. ABV does not taste very good and does not deliver as much stimulation as fresh buds do. People generally prefer vaporizing cannabis because it does not combust the herb, and obviously smoking ABV totally defeats this purpose. However, you can still get slight stimulation from smoking ABV.

2) Direct Approach
If you prefer ingesting the plant material directly, you can sprinkle ABV buds (only a fraction of an ounce) onto your pizzas, sandwiches and pastas, or into your smoothies and drinks. ABV tastes very similar to fresh buds with almost the same aroma, but with a little more "toasted" flavor.

3) ABV Coconut Oil
This works great for your favorite pastas, snacks and salad dressings. Over low heat, mix a pint of coconut oil and half an ounce of ABV in a saucepan until they are incorporated. Optionally, you can use soy lecithin to bind everything together. Strain the oil and store it in the refrigerator for later use.

4) Cannabutter
Cannabutter is quite popular and has been used in hundreds of cannabis-infused recipes. Use ABV and butter in a 1:1 ratio to make cannabutter. The quantity of water needed depends on the volume of the ingredients; use adequate water to cover the ingredients in a saucepan. You can find the recipe on page 13.

Why it is Important to Decarboxylate Cannabis

In its raw form, the cannabis plant is non-psychoactive. It only becomes psychoactive when the buds dry out, when they age, or when they are heated. Heating activates more psychoactive compounds than aging. In order to release the maximum potential of the plant's psychoactive compounds, the decarboxylating or "decarbing" process must be completed.

Decarboxylation Process

1. Preheat oven to 240°F.
2. Break cannabis buds and flowers into smaller bits using your hands.
3. Arrange the pieces in a single layer on a medium-sized baking pan lined with parchment paper.
4. The cannabis should cover the pan completely so that there is no empty space on the sheet.
5. Bake the buds for 35–40 minutes. Stir two or three times in between for even toasting.
6. After the buds dry out and darken, remove the pan from the oven and let it cool for 20–25 minutes. The texture should be crumbly.
7. In a food processor, process the buds until they are coarsely ground. Be careful you do not over-process and turn the cannabis into powder.
8. Store in an airtight glass container.
9. Follow the same process for decarbing kief and stems. (Dried resin buds, collected from cannabis plant leaves, are used to make kief. These buds can be ground to make fine powder, which is known as "kief".)

Decarboxylated Cannabis-Infused Oil

Decarboxylated cannabis (prepared as above) is used to make cannabis-infused oil. Pick an oil that has a high fat content and is made from an unmodified, natural crop. Oils with low heating points are best, as they preserve the original taste of the oil after the cannabis flavor is infused. Below are some recommended oils to use for cannabis infusion:

1) Olive Oil
Olive oil is incredibly healthy, natural, and flavorful. It is perfectly suited for salad dressings, flatbread pizza, pastas, or as a dip to use with your favorite bread.

Use high-quality extra virgin olive oil made from natural, real olives and not the colored or repackaged versions of vegetable oils.

2) Coconut Oil
Coconut oil is one of the most recommended choices for preparing cannabis-infused oil because it contains the highest saturated fat content. It thus absorbs more cannabinoids than other oils. It also has a better shelf life when processed or heated.

Making Cannabutter or
Cannabis Butter at Home

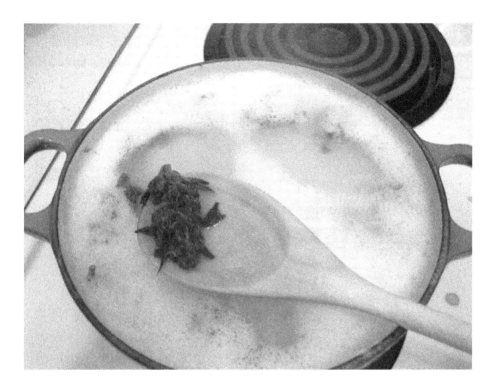

Ingredients
1 cup water
1 pound unsalted butter
1 ounce cannabis, coarsely ground

Directions
1. Place the unsalted butter and water in a stockpot or saucepan.
2. Gradually warm the pot over low heat.
3. Let the butter melt and bring it to a simmer to completely melt the butter into the water.
4. Stir the flower into the mixture.

5. Simmer for 2½–3 hours, stirring occasionally. Do not let the mixture boil.
6. Pour the mixture into a glass container with a tight-fitting lid.
7. Use a piece of cheesecloth or a fine metal strainer to filter out the plant material from the prepared mix.
8. Squeeze the cheesecloth to extract all the liquid. Discard the remaining plant material.
9. Cool for 10–15 minutes.
10. Cover and store the cannabutter in the refrigerator for 10–12 hours to harden.
11. The hardened butter will separate from the water so you can easily take it out and use it in your recipes.
12. Discard the remaining water.
13. Store the cannabutter at room temperature if you will use it soon.
14. You can also store it in the freezer for later use. The butter stays good for 2–3 months when stored in a freezer. When you're ready to use it, take it out and let it thaw at room temperature for 15–20 minutes before using. (There is no need to warm it up in a microwave or oven.)

Making Cannabis Oil at Home

Ingredients
1⅖ ounces decarboxylated cannabis
2 cups unrefined coconut oil

Directions
1. Mix the coconut oil and cannabis in a saucepan. Gradually warm it over low heat.
2. Simmer the mixture for 50–60 minutes, stirring occasionally. Do not cover the pan.
3. Place a metal strainer lined with cheesecloth over a bowl to filter out the cannabis particles.
4. Pour the mixture into the strainer and allow it to drip for about 60–75 minutes.
5. Wrap the plant material in the cheesecloth and squeeze out any leftover liquid. Discard the solids.
6. Cool the liquid mixture in a glass container for 10–15 minutes and allow it to solidify.
7. Cover the container and place it in the refrigerator. The oil is usually good for up to 10–12 months.

Making Canna-cream or Canna-milk at Home

Ingredients

½ ounce decarboxylated cannabis, finely crumbled
1¼ cups of your choice of heavy whipping cream, whole milk, almond milk or coconut milk

Directions

1. Fill a deep saucepan with water and simmer it.
2. Fold up a kitchen towel and place it in the bottom of the saucepan.
3. Add the milk and crumbled cannabis to a wide mouth 16-ounce canning jar such as a Mason jar. Close the lid and place the jar in the simmering water over the folded towel. The water should cover tree quarter of the jar.
4. Simmer for 80–90 minutes, topping up the water as needed.
5. Take the jar out of the water every 20 minutes with tongs and pot holders and carefully open the lid to stir the milk with a wooden spoon and release pressure.
6. Cool down completely and store in an airtight container in your fridge up to 3–5 days.

Being Safe while Infusing

- If possible, infuse oils outside in the open air to minimize the risk of fire or explosion. If you are inside, open the windows and start a fan for better air circulation.
- If you have a respiratory condition or sensitive lungs, use a facemask.
- Make sure that you are using proper equipment. While preparing an infusion that involves solvents, a double boiler pot and pan setup is better, with the solvent pan being on top of the water pot, and not directly on the heating element of the stove. Follow this precaution with both gas and electric stoves. Always wear a face mask when working with solvents.
- To avoid unexpected hazards, prepare canna infusion oil when there are minimum distractions and you're not in a hurry.
- Be more alert when preparing infusion oil or butter on a gas stove. Avoid placing the solvent pan near the stove when the flame is on, as it can catch fire.
- Once you're finished making canna oil or butter, be sure to turn off the oven, the stove and any other open flame heating element.
- Store your oils and edibles in child-resistant containers in a dry place that is difficult for children and pets to reach. Accidental ingestion of cannabis-infused oil by children and pets may lead to many health issues.

Breakfast & Smoothies

Cranberry Granola Breakfast

Serves: 6
Preparation time: 5–8 minutes
Cooking time: 35 minutes

Ingredients
1½ cups rolled oats
⅓ cup sweetened coconut flakes
¼ cup hemp seeds, hulled
¼ cup honey
¾ cup dried cranberries
⅓ cup sliced almonds
1 egg white
2 tablespoons cannabis-coconut oil
2 tablespoons coconut oil
¼ teaspoon cinnamon
⅛ teaspoon salt

Directions
1. Preheat oven to 300°F or 148°C. Line a large baking sheet with parchment paper.
2. In a medium-large mixing bowl, thoroughly combine the oats, cranberries, almonds, coconut flakes and hemp seeds.
3. In another bowl, whisk together the honey, both oils, egg white, cinnamon and salt.
4. Add this mixture over the oat mixture and combine well.
5. Spread the oat mixture over the prepared baking sheet to make a thin layer.
6. Bake for about 35 minutes or until browned.
7. Stir the mixture every 8–10 minutes.
8. Serve warm.

Nutrition (per serving)
Calories 356
Carbs 42.3g, Fat 19g, Protein 7.2g, Sodium 72mg

Mushroom Egg Omelet Morning

Serves: 1–2
Preparation time: 5 minutes
Cooking time: 10 minutes

Ingredients
½ teaspoon canna-coconut oil
2 tablespoons onion, finely diced
2 tablespoons bell pepper, finely diced
2 eggs
½ teaspoon cannabutter
1 small tomato, diced
2 ounces Cremini mushrooms
1 teaspoon flaxseed
Ground black pepper and salt, to taste

Directions
1. Heat the canna-coconut oil over medium heat in a medium skillet or saucepan.
2. Add the onions and stir gently; cook while stirring until translucent and softened.
3. Add the bell peppers and mushrooms; cook while stirring until tender.
4. Add the tomatoes and cook for 1–2 minutes. Set aside to cool.
5. Melt the cannabutter in the skillet or saucepan.
6. Crack the eggs in, spread to make a circle, and season to taste.
7. Add the flaxseed and cook until fluffy.
8. Add the vegetable mix over half; fold the omelet and serve.

Nutrition (per serving)
Calories 204
Carbs 3.6g, Fat 17.4g, Protein 8g, Sodium 81mg

Apple Cinnamon Pancakes

Serves: 8–10
Preparation time: 10 minutes
Cooking time: 15–20 minutes

Ingredients
1 teaspoon salt
2 cups milk
2 cups almond flour
3 tablespoons baking powder
½ cup + 2 tablespoons canna-coconut oil
2 apples, peeled, cored and shredded
2 eggs, beaten
2 large carrots, peeled and shredded
2 tablespoons vanilla extract
1 teaspoon cinnamon

Directions
1. Combine the flour, baking powder and salt in a mixing bowl.
2. Combine the milk, cinnamon, carrot, apple, vanilla extract, eggs and ½ cup canna-coconut oil in a separate bowl.
3. Mix both the mixtures with each other.
4. Heat the 2 tablespoons of canna-coconut oil in a medium skillet or saucepan over medium heat.
5. Add ½ cup of batter and spread to make a circle. Cook on both sides until golden brown.
6. Repeat with the remaining batter.
7. Serve warm.

Nutrition (per serving)
Calories 219
Carbs 15.3g, Fat 16.1g, Protein 4.6g, Sodium 344mg

Avocado Toast

Serves: 4
Preparation time: 10 minutes
Cooking time: 0 minutes

Ingredients
1 ripe medium avocado
1 teaspoon balsamic vinegar
4 slices sourdough bread, toasted
8 tomato slices
8 slices bacon, cooked
Pinch of finely crumbled, decarboxylated kief or buds
Freshly ground black pepper and salt to taste

Directions
1. Halve the avocado, remove the pit, and scoop out the flesh.
2. In a mixing bowl, combine the avocado flesh, crumbled kief or bud, balsamic vinegar, black pepper and salt.
3. Spread the prepared mix over the toast slices.
4. Arrange 2 tomato slices and 2 bacon slices over each slice.

Nutrition (per serving)
Calories 263
Carbs 27.6g, Fat 13g, Protein 10.2g, Sodium 323mg

Banana Bread

Serves: 12–14 slices
Preparation time: 10 minutes
Cooking time: 25 minutes

Ingredients
½ teaspoon baking powder
½ teaspoon baking soda
¼ cup sugar
¼ cup packed brown sugar
½ teaspoon salt
¾ cup all-purpose flour
½ cup whole-wheat flour
½ teaspoon nutmeg
4 medium-size mashed bananas
¼ cup buttermilk
¼ cup cannabutter, melted
2 tablespoons honey
1 large egg
1 teaspoon vanilla extract
Cooking spray

Directions
1. Preheat oven to 350°F or 176°C.
2. Grease an 8×4-inch bread pan with cooking spray.
3. In a mixing bowl, combine the all-purpose flour, whole-wheat flour, salt, sugar, brown sugar, baking powder, baking soda and nutmeg.
4. In another large bowl, combine the mashed bananas, buttermilk, cannabutter, honey, egg and vanilla extract; mix well.
5. Mix the flour mix with the egg mix to make a dough-like consistency.

6. Add the mix to the bread pan; bake for 20–25 until the bread has risen and a toothpick inserted comes out dry.
7. Let the pan cool before removing the loaf.
8. Shake the pan and take out the loaf. Slice and serve.

Nutrition (per slice)
Calories 116
Carbs 18.6g, Fat 4.1g, Protein 2.2g, Sodium 181mg

Cannabis Pancakes

Serves: 2
Preparation time: 8–10 minutes
Cooking time: 25 minutes

Ingredients
Juice of ½ lemon
2 tablespoons confectioners' sugar
1 tablespoon canna-milk or canna-cream
1 tablespoon sugar
½ teaspoon salt
⅛ teaspoon ground nutmeg (optional)
¾ cup whole milk
¾ cup all-purpose flour
3 eggs
¼ cup unsalted butter, melted

Directions
1. In a medium-large mixing bowl, thoroughly whisk the whole milk, canna-milk or canna-cream, flour, eggs, sugar, salt and nutmeg until no lumps are visible.
2. Melt the butter over medium heat in a large skillet or saucepan.
3. Add the batter and spread to make a circle.
4. Cook on both sides until golden brown.
5. Transfer to a serving plate and divide into two parts; top with the lemon juice and sugar and serve warm.

Nutrition (per serving)
Calories 411
Carbs 38.4g, Fat 22.7g, Protein 12.6g, Sodium 456mg

Lamb Egg Omelet

Serves: 1–2
Preparation time: 5 minutes
Cooking time: 8–10 minutes

Ingredients
1 clove garlic, minced
1 ounce ground lamb
1 teaspoon mint
1 teaspoon cannabutter
1 tablespoon fennel, diced
3 rainbow chards, wilted
3 eggs
Ground black pepper and salt to taste

Directions
1. Whisk the eggs in a mixing bowl; season to taste.
2. In a medium skillet or saucepan, melt the cannabutter over medium heat.
3. Add the beaten eggs and cook for 10 seconds. Add the garlic, ground lamb, fennel and rainbow chard.
4. Cook until the lamb is evenly brown and the omelet is cooked well.
5. Serve warm with the mint on top.

Nutrition (per serving)
Calories 307
Carbs 14.2g, Fat 8.3g, Protein 10.4g, Sodium 172mg

Cafe Mocha

Serves: 1
Preparation time: 8–10 minutes
Cooking time: 5 minutes

Ingredients
2 tablespoons chocolate syrup
¾ cup freshly brewed hot coffee
¾ cup whole milk
1½ teaspoons canna-milk or canna-cream
Whipped cream (optional)

Directions:
1. To a medium skillet or saucepan, add both the milks and heat over medium heat. Do not boil.
2. To a coffee mug, add the hot milk and chocolate syrup.
3. Combine well. Add the coffee and stir gently.
4. Top with the cream.

Nutrition (per serving)
Calories 233
Carbs 28.4g, Fat 7.3g, Protein 7.4g, Sodium 148mg

Strawberry Smoothie

Serves: 5–6
Preparation time: 10 minutes
Cooking time: 3–4 minutes

Ingredients

3 tablespoons canna-coconut oil
2 bananas, frozen and sliced
3 cups coconut milk
3 cups strawberries, frozen
3 tablespoons pomegranate molasses
⅜ cup pomegranate juice
Ice cubes (optional)

Directions

1. To a medium skillet or saucepan, add the canna-coconut oil and heat it over medium heat.
2. Add the banana slices and cook for 3–4 minutes. Let cool completely.
3. To a food processor or blender, add the bananas and remaining ingredients.
4. Blend or process on pulse mode until you get a smooth mixture.
5. Add to a smoothie glass and serve.

Nutrition (per serving)

Calories 187
Carbs 19.3g, Fat 9.2g, Protein 3g, Sodium 22mg

Choco Smoothie

Serves: 2
Preparation time: 5 minutes
Cooking time: 0 minutes

Ingredients
½ cup cold water
3 bananas, frozen and sliced
1 cup almond milk
2–3 tablespoons chocolate syrup, or more to taste
2 tablespoons cannabutter
¼ teaspoon almond extract
2 tablespoons cocoa powder, unsweetened
Ice cubes (optional)

Directions
1. To a food processor or blender, add the water, milk and remaining ingredients except the cocoa powder.
2. Blend or process on pulse mode until you get a smooth mixture.
3. Add to a smoothie glass, top with the cocoa powder, and serve.

Nutrition (per serving)
Calories 445
Carbs 48.5g, Fat 14.4g, Protein 5.3g, Sodium 208mg

Banana Smoothie

Serves: 2
Preparation time: 5 minutes
Cooking time: 0 minutes

Ingredients
⅓ cup low-fat vanilla yogurt
2 cups almond milk
3 tablespoons honey
¼ cup peanut butter
2 tablespoons canna-coconut oil
1 teaspoon vanilla
¼ cup oatmeal
2 bananas, frozen and sliced
Ice cubes (optional)

Directions
1. To a food processor or blender, add the milk, yogurt and remaining ingredients.
2. Blend or process on pulse mode until you get a smooth mixture.
3. Add to a smoothie glass and serve.

Nutrition (per serving)
Calories 407
Carbs 36.5g, Fat 13.4g, Protein 7.1g, Sodium 214mg

Savory Recipes

Broccoli Cream Soup

Serves: 3–4
Preparation time: 15 minutes
Cooking time: 10–15 minutes

Ingredients
1 cup broccoli florets, chopped
1 cup celery, chopped
2 cups heavy cream
¼ cup yellow onions, diced
1 tablespoon flour
3 cups vegetable stock
¼ cup cannabutter

Directions
1. Heat the vegetable stock in a cooking pot over medium heat.
2. In a saucepan, melt the cannabutter over medium heat.
3. Add the onions and celery and cook while stirring until softened for 4–5 minutes.
4. Mix in the flour and add the mix to the cooking pot.
5. Stir the mixture and simmer over low heat.
6. Add the broccoli florets and simmer until softened and cooked well.
7. Mix in the cream and simmer for 1–2 minutes.
8. Serve warm.

Nutrition (per serving)
Calories 456
Carbs 7.6g, Fat 23.6g, Protein 3.4g, Sodium 81mg

Chicken Lettuce Wraps

Serves: 4
Preparation time: 10 minutes
Cooking time: 25 minutes

Ingredients
1 ounce mushrooms, finely diced
1 clove garlic, minced
4 lettuce leaves
1 pound ground chicken
1 tablespoon cannabis-olive oil
1 tablespoon vinegar
Salt to taste

Directions
1. To a medium skillet or saucepan, add the cannabis-olive oil and heat it over medium heat.
2. Add the chicken and stir gently; cook while stirring for 8–10 minutes until evenly brown.
3. Add the mushroom and cook for 8–10 minutes.
4. Add the vinegar and garlic; combine well.
5. Season with salt and cook for 4–5 minutes.
6. Add the mix over the lettuce leaves evenly; wrap and serve.

Nutrition (per serving)
Calories 234
Carbs 2g, Fat 11.3g, Protein 21.4g, Sodium 97mg

Cannabis Mayonnaise

Serves/Yield: ¾ cup
Preparation time: 5 minutes
Cooking time: 0 minutes

Ingredients
1 teaspoon Dijon mustard
¾ cup vegetable oil
¼ cup cannabis-coconut oil
2 egg yolks
4 teaspoons lemon juice
Ground black pepper and salt to taste

Directions
1. Add the egg yolks, lemon juice and mustard to a blender or food processor.
2. Blend until well combined.
3. Drizzle in the vegetable oil and cannabis-coconut oil.
4. Blend until thick.
5. Season with ground black pepper and salt.
6. Refrigerate in an airtight container; use within 48 hours.

Nutrition (per tablespoon)
Calories 121
Carbs 6.3g, Fat 12.5g, Protein 0.2g, Sodium 13mg

Bone Broth

Serves: 3–4
Preparation time: 3–5 minutes
Cooking time: 4–6 hours

Ingredients
3–4 fish carcasses (halibut, turbot, rockfish, or snapper), with heads, without oil
2 tablespoons cannabutter
1 carrot, chopped
2 onions, chopped
Dry thyme and dry parsley as required
½ cup dry white wine
1 bay leaf
¼ cup apple cider vinegar
3 quarts water

Directions
1. To a medium-large cooking pot or deep saucepan, add the cannabutter and melt it over medium heat.
2. Add the vegetables and stir gently; cook while stirring until softened.
3. Add the white wine and bring to a boil. Add the fish and fill the pot with water.
4. Mix in the vinegar and bring to a boil again. Discard any fat that surfaces.
5. Add thyme and parsley and reduce heat to low.
6. Cover and cook for 4–6 hours.
7. Let the liquid cool down, then strain it into jars.
8. Refrigerate for later use.

Nutrition (per serving)
Calories 90
Carbs 3.6g, Fat 7.6g, Protein 4.3g, Sodium 52mg

Cheesy Mushroom Soup

Serves: 4–5
Preparation time: 5–8 minutes
Cooking time: 20 minutes

Ingredients
2 cloves garlic, peeled and minced
2 cups water
2 tablespoons balsamic vinegar
3 cups mushrooms, cleaned and sliced
3 cups chicken broth
2 medium onions, peeled and sliced thinly
3 tablespoons cannabutter
½ cup tomato paste
3 tablespoons parsley, chopped
1 teaspoon salt
½ teaspoon ground black pepper
½ cup parmesan cheese, shredded

Directions
1. In a medium skillet or saucepan, melt the cannabutter over medium heat.
2. Add the onions and garlic and stir gently; cook while stirring until translucent and softened.
3. Add the mushrooms; cover and cook for 4–5 minutes.
4. Add the chicken broth, tomato paste, water, balsamic vinegar, salt and pepper; stir to mix.
5. Bring to a boil and lower the heat; cover and cook for another 8–10 minutes.
6. Top with the shredded parmesan and parsley; serve warm.

Nutrition (per serving)
Calories 269
Carbs 12.6g, Fat 15.7g, Protein 19.4g, Sodium 978mg

Cheesy Lettuce Bacon Salad

Serves: 4
Preparation time: 10–15 minutes
Cooking time: 0 minutes

Ingredients
1 tablespoon lemon juice
4 ounces crumbled blue cheese
⅜ cup sour cream
1 tablespoon cannabis mayonnaise
2 tablespoons chives, chopped
1 head iceberg lettuce, quartered
4 slices bacon, cooked and crumbled
½ teaspoon ground black pepper
¼ teaspoon salt
2 large tomatoes, seeded and diced
2 medium avocados, peeled, pitted and diced

Directions
1. In a mixing bowl, whisk the sour cream, cannabis mayonnaise and lemon juice.
2. Mix in the blue cheese, chives, black pepper and salt.
3. Arrange the lettuce quarters on 4 plates.
4. Drizzle the dressing over them; top with the crumbled bacon, tomatoes and avocado; serve warm.

Nutrition (per serving)
Calories 259
Carbs 9.6g, Fat 23.4g, Protein 8.4g, Sodium 522mg

Bacon Potato Salad

Serves: 4–5
Preparation time: 5 minutes
Cooking time: 15–20 minutes

Ingredients
3 scallions, chopped
¼ cup cannabis-olive oil
2 pounds potatoes, peeled and cubed
6 cherry tomatoes, halved
5 strips bacon, cooked
½ cup snap peas, raw
½ teaspoon dill, chopped

Directions
1. To a medium skillet or saucepan, add the cannabis-olive oil and heat it over medium heat.
2. Add the scallions and stir gently; cook while stirring until softened.
3. Add the tomatoes and cook for 2–3 minutes.
4. Add the remaining ingredients; cook while stirring until the potatoes are soft.
5. Top with the chopped dill and serve.

Nutrition (per serving)
Calories 254
Carbs 38.6g, Fat 5.1g, Protein 9.6g, Sodium 154mg

Broccoli Beef Meal

Serves: 4–5
Preparation time: 5 minutes
Cooking time: 10–15 minutes

Ingredients

1 cup onion, minced
2 cups broccoli, chopped
1 pound beef, cut into small pieces
2 tablespoons cannabis-coconut oil
1 tablespoon sesame seeds
3 tablespoons green onion, chopped
1 cup chestnuts, sliced (optional)

Directions

1. In a medium skillet or saucepan, heat the cannabis-coconut oil over medium heat.
2. Add the beef cubes and stir gently; cook while stirring until evenly brown. Set aside.
3. Add the onions and broccoli and stir gently; cook while stirring until the onions soften and the broccoli wilts.
4. Add the cooked beef and cook while stirring for 2–3 minutes.
5. Top with the sesame seeds, green onion and chestnuts.

Nutrition (per serving)

Calories 359
Carbs 11.4g, Fat 28.7g, Protein 12.6g, Sodium 874mg

Kale Bacon Meal

Serves: 5–6
Preparation time: 5 minutes
Cooking time: 20–25 minutes

Ingredients
4 cloves garlic, minced
6 slices bacon, raw
2 large bunches kale leaves
2 cups onions, chopped
¼ cup cannabutter
1 tablespoon sesame seeds, roasted
½ teaspoon pecans, chopped

Directions
1. In a medium skillet or saucepan, melt the cannabutter over medium heat.
2. Add the bacon strips and stir gently; cook while stirring to crisp. Reserve the fat in the saucepan and set aside the cooked bacon.
3. Add the onion and sauté until translucent. Add the garlic; cook while stirring for 1 minute.
4. Add the kale leaves and cook while stirring until wilted and softened.
5. Add the bacon and gently mix.
6. Garnish with the sesame seeds and pecans; serve warm.

Nutrition (per serving)
Calories 366
Carbs 14.6g, Fat 27.5g, Protein 9.3g, Sodium 188mg

Bacon Spinach Stir-Fry

Serves: 2–3
Preparation time: 8–10 minutes
Cooking time: 20 minutes

Ingredients

¼ cup shallots, chopped
¼ pound raw bacon slices, chopped
1 tablespoon cannabutter
½ pound raw spinach
¼ cup white onion, chopped

Directions

1. In a medium skillet or saucepan, melt the cannabutter over medium heat.
2. Add the onions, shallots and bacon and stir gently; cook while stirring for 12–15 minutes until the bacon is crisp and brown and the onions are softened.
3. Add the spinach leaves and cook while stirring until wilted.
4. Serve warm.

Nutrition (per serving)

Calories 113
Carbs 5.3g, Fat 9.8g, Protein 1.4g, Sodium 18mg

Lamb Mayo Salad

Serves: 2–3
Preparation time: 10–15 minutes
Cooking time: 18–20 minutes

Ingredients
Salad
1 cup tomato, sliced
½ cup green onion, sliced
2 tablespoons cannabis olive oil
1 cup lamb, diced
½ cup celery, diced

Dressing
¼ teaspoon thyme, dried
¼ teaspoon tarragon, dried
1 ounce cream cheese, softened
1 ounce mayonnaise
1 tablespoon honey
Ground black pepper and salt to taste

Directions
Dressing
1. In a mixing bowl, whisk the cream cheese, honey and mayonnaise to make a smooth mix.
2. Season to taste and mix in the thyme and tarragon.

Salad
1. To a medium skillet or saucepan, add the cannabis olive oil and heat it over medium heat.
2. Add the onions and celery and stir gently; cook while stirring for 8–10 minutes until translucent and softened.
3. Add the diced lamb and cook for 13–15 minutes or until cooked well.

4. Transfer the mixture to a serving bowl; mix in the tomato and top with the dressing.
5. Toss well and serve.

Nutrition (per serving)
Calories 346
Carbs 15.3g, Fat 14g, Protein 37.8g, Sodium 117mg

Bulgur Salad

Serves: 4
Preparation time: 20–25 minutes
Cooking time: 0 minutes

Ingredients
¾ cup Italian parsley, chopped
¼ cup mint, chopped
1½ teaspoons salt
1½ cups ripe tomatoes, diced and seeded
¾ cup scallions, minced
1⅓ cups boiling water
¾ cup dry bulgur wheat
5 tablespoons lemon juice
3 tablespoons extra-virgin olive oil
1 tablespoon cannabis olive oil
2 teaspoons minced garlic
Ground black pepper to taste

Directions
1. Mix the boiling water, bulgur and salt in a large mixing bowl. Cover and set aside for 15 minutes or until the bulgur turns soft and the water is absorbed.
2. Mix in the tomatoes, scallions, parsley, mint, lemon juice, olive oil, cannabis olive oil and garlic.
3. Combine well and season to taste. Serve.

Nutrition (per serving)
Calories 276
Carbs 38.4g, Fat 11.2g, Protein 11.4g, Sodium 651mg

Parmesan Pasta

Serves: 5–6
Preparation time: 10–15 minutes
Cooking time: 15–20 minutes

Ingredients
4 cloves garlic, roughly chopped
1 pound angel hair pasta
¼ cup cannabutter
Ground black pepper and salt, to taste
¼ cup parsley, chopped
¾ cup parmesan cheese, shredded

Directions
1. Cook the pasta in salted water in a saucepan as per the package instructions.
2. Drain the water and set aside the pasta.
3. In a medium skillet or saucepan, melt the cannabutter over medium heat.
4. Add the parsley and garlic and stir gently; cook while stirring until translucent and softened.
5. Mix in the pasta and season to taste; combine well.
6. Top with the parmesan cheese and serve.

Nutrition (per serving)
Calories 346
Carbs 54.6g, Fat 12.6g, Protein 13g, Sodium 134mg

Chicken Spinach Tortillas

Serves: 4
Preparation time: 10 minutes
Cooking time: 15–20 minutes

Ingredients
1 pound chicken, cubed
4 (10-inch) flour tortillas, cooked
4 cups raw spinach
½ cup shallots, chopped
1 tablespoon cannabutter

Directions
1. In a medium skillet or saucepan, melt the cannabutter over medium heat.
2. Add the shallots and chicken and stir gently; cook while stirring until the shallots are softened and the chicken is evenly brown.
3. Add the spinach and cook while stirring until wilted.
4. Transfer the mixture onto the tortillas and roll them up.
5. Serve with a dip of your choice.

Nutrition (per serving)
Calories 253
Carbs 23.4g, Fat 7g, Protein 26.4g, Sodium 344mg

Chicken Curry

Serves: 4
Preparation time: 10–15 minutes
Cooking time: 25 minutes

Ingredients
1 jalapeno pepper, cored, seeded and minced
1 tablespoon cannabis coconut oil
1 tablespoon curry powder
½ cup plain yogurt
½ cup chicken stock
2 teaspoons grated ginger
1½ teaspoons garlic, minced
2 tablespoons extra-virgin olive oil
1½ pounds boneless, skinless chicken breasts, cubed
1 large onion, diced
½ teaspoon turmeric
¼ cup cilantro, minced
Ground black pepper and salt to taste

Directions
1. To a medium skillet or saucepan, add the olive oil and heat it over medium heat.
2. Add the onions, chicken and jalapeno and stir gently; cook while stirring for 4–5 minutes until the onions soften and the chicken is evenly brown.
3. Stir in the curry powder, ginger, garlic, cannabis coconut oil and turmeric and mix until well combined.
4. Reduce heat to medium-low. Add the yogurt and cook while stirring for 2–3 minutes until thickened.
5. Stir in the chicken stock and cilantro. Season to taste.
6. Reduce heat to low; cover and simmer, stirring occasionally, for about 15 minutes or until the chicken is well cooked.
7. Serve warm.

Nutrition (per serving)
Calories 195
Carbs 4.2g, Fat 13.4g, Protein 12.6g, Sodium 76mg

Creamy Coleslaw

Serves: 5–6
Preparation time: 8–10 minutes
Cooking time: 0 minutes

Ingredients
1 tablespoon Dijon mustard
1 tablespoon lemon juice
1 teaspoon sugar
½ cup cannabis mayonnaise
¼ cup mayonnaise
Ground black pepper and salt to taste
2 cups shredded coleslaw mix (carrots, red cabbage and green cabbage)

Directions
1. In a medium-large mixing bowl, thoroughly combine the mayonnaise, cannabis mayonnaise, mustard, lemon juice and sugar. Season with black pepper and salt.
2. Add the coleslaw mix and toss to coat well.
3. Serve fresh or refrigerate to chill and serve cold.

Nutrition (per serving)
Calories 76
Carbs 4.3g, Fat 7.4g, Protein 0.4g, Sodium 71mg

Chicken Wings

Serves: 4–5
Preparation time: 8–10 minutes
Cooking time: 15–20 minutes

Ingredients
2 pounds chicken wings
3 tablespoons vegetable oil
½ cup red hot sauce
½ cup cannabutter
Ranch dressing or dip of your choice, to serve

Directions
1. To a medium skillet or saucepan, add the vegetable oil and heat it over medium heat.
2. Add the chicken wings and stir gently; cook while stirring until evenly golden brown.
3. Transfer to a serving plate.
4. In another saucepan, melt the cannabutter.
5. Add the hot sauce and mix well. Set aside.
6. Top the wings with the cannabutter sauce and coat well.
7. Serve with the ranch dressing or dip of your choice.

Nutrition (per serving)
Calories 453
Carbs 5.3g, Fat 34.6g, Protein 24.6g, Sodium 1123mg

Shrimp Creole

Serves: 4
Preparation time: 8–10 minutes
Cooking time: 35 minutes

Ingredients
2 tablespoons all-purpose flour
½ small onion, diced
½ small green bell pepper, cored and diced
1 large celery rib, finely diced
2 teaspoons garlic, minced
1 tablespoon unsalted butter, melted
1 tablespoon extra-virgin olive oil
2 cups tomatoes, crushed
1 cup chicken or vegetable stock
1 bay leaf
⅛ teaspoon cayenne pepper
2 tablespoons chopped Italian parsley
1 tablespoon cannabis coconut or cannabis olive oil
Salt to taste
1 pound medium shrimp, peeled and deveined
Cooked rice, to serve

Directions
1. To a medium skillet or saucepan, add the olive oil and heat it over medium heat.
2. Add the butter and then mix in the flour; whisk thoroughly.
3. Cook while stirring for 3–4 minutes to form roux.
4. Add the onion, bell pepper and celery; cook while stirring for 3–4 minutes until softened.
5. Stir in the garlic and cook for 1 minute more.
6. Stir in the tomatoes and their juices, stock, cannabis coconut or cannabis olive oil, bay leaf, cayenne, parsley and salt.

7. Increase heat and bring the mixture to a boil.
8. Reduce heat and simmer for about 15 minutes.
9. Add the shrimp; cook while stirring for 4–5 minutes until the shrimp are no longer translucent.
10. Take out the bay leaf and serve over the cooked rice.

Nutrition (per serving)
Calories 286
Carbs 34.6g, Fat 8.1g, Protein 36.4g, Sodium 546mg

Grilled Steak

Serves: 6
Preparation time: 8–10 minutes
Cooking time: 10 minutes

Ingredients

1¼ cups Italian parsley
2 tablespoons cannabis olive oil
⅔ cup extra-virgin olive oil
⅓ cup lemon juice
½ teaspoon crushed red pepper
1½ pounds flank steak
2 tablespoons minced garlic
1 teaspoon salt plus more to season
1 teaspoon ground black pepper plus more to season

Directions

1. Preheat a grill to medium heat.
2. Add the parsley, cannabis olive oil, olive oil, lemon juice, garlic, 1 teaspoon salt, 1 teaspoon black pepper and red pepper to a blender or food processor.
3. Blend to make a puree. Set aside.
4. Season the steak evenly with salt and black pepper.
5. Grill the steak for 4–5 minutes per side until cooked to preferred doneness.
6. Remove the steak, let cool, and slice it.
7. Top with the puree and serve warm.

Nutrition (per serving)

Calories 233
Carbs 2.3g, Fat 17.6g, Protein 3.6g, Sodium 348mg

Tomato Jalapeno Soup

Serves: 5–6
Preparation time: 8–10 minutes
Cooking time: 0 minutes

Ingredients
¼ cup red wine vinegar
2 jalapeno peppers, cored, seeded and minced (optional)
5 ripe tomatoes, chopped
1 medium cucumber, peeled, seeded and chopped
1 medium yellow or red bell pepper, chopped
1 (12-ounce) can tomato juice
2 tablespoons Italian parsley or cilantro, minced
2 tablespoons cannabis olive oil
1 tablespoon extra-virgin olive oil
1 teaspoon garlic, minced
Ground black pepper and salt to taste

Directions
1. To a mixing bowl, add the pepper, cucumber and tomatoes.
2. Add the tomato juice, parsley, red wine vinegar, jalapeno, cannabis oil, olive oil and garlic.
3. Combine to mix well.
4. Season to taste and mix again.
5. Serve and enjoy.

Nutrition (per serving)
Calories 103
Carbs 13.6g, Fat 3.4g, Protein 2.8g, Sodium 178mg

Caesar Salad

Serves: 4
Preparation time: 15 minutes
Cooking time: 0 minutes

Ingredients
Dressing
1 tablespoon lemon juice
1½ teaspoons Worcestershire sauce
¾ teaspoon Dijon mustard
½ teaspoon garlic, minced
1 can of 4 anchovy fillets with oil
1 egg yolk
¼ cup extra-virgin olive oil
1 tablespoon cannabis olive oil
Ground black pepper and salt to taste

Salad
¾ cup croutons
24 romaine lettuce leaves
¼ cup parmesan cheese, shredded

Directions
Dressing
1. To a blender or food processor, add the anchovy fillets, egg yolk, lemon juice, Worcestershire sauce, mustard and garlic.
2. Blend to make a smooth mix.
3. Drizzle in the olive oil and cannabis olive oil.
4. Continue to blend to emulsify. Season to taste.

Salad

1. Arrange the romaine leaves on plates.
2. Drizzle with the dressing; top with the croutons and parmesan cheese.
3. Serve fresh.

Nutrition (per serving)

Calories 368

Carbs 28.6g, Fat 31.3g, Protein 23.6g, Sodium 854mg

Spiced Iced Tea

Serves: 9–10
Preparation time: 10–15 minutes
Cooking time: 0 minutes

Ingredients
1 teaspoon vanilla extract
2¼ quarts boiling water
7 tea bags of your choice, such as Darjeeling or English Breakfast
1 teaspoon cinnamon
2 pods cardamom
2 star anise
1 cup granulated sugar (optional)
5 tablespoons cannabutter, melted
2¼ cups condensed milk

Directions
1. Arrange the tea bags in a large tea pot and pour in the boiling water.
2. Steep for 4–5 minutes. Remove the tea bags.
3. To a pitcher, add the prepared tea, spices and sugar. Let cool to room temperature.
4. Mix the cannabutter and condensed milk in a bowl and whisk well.
5. Refrigerate both the milk mixture and the prepared tea.
6. Pour the tea into glasses and add ¼ cup of the milk mixture to each; stir.
7. Serve chilled.

Nutrition (per serving)
Calories 268
Carbs 32.3g, Fat 6.2g, Protein 5.4g, Sodium 78mg

Snacks

Cheesy Kale Chips

Serves: 6
Preparation time: 5 minutes
Baking time: 25 minutes

Ingredients
¾ pound kale leaves, stemmed
⅓ cup parmesan cheese, grated
2 tablespoons cannabis olive oil
2 teaspoons ground black pepper

Directions
1. Preheat oven to 250°F or 120°C. Line a medium baking sheet with parchment paper.
2. Place the kale leaves in a mixing bowl, drizzle with the cannabis olive oil and toss to coat.
3. Sprinkle with the black pepper and top with the cheese; combine well.
4. Arrange over the baking sheet. Do not overcrowd.
5. Bake for about 25 minutes or until crisp, shaking the baking sheet several times during cooking.
6. Serve warm.

Nutrition (per serving)
Calories 107
Carbs 3.3g, Fat 6.4g, Protein 9.4g, Sodium 376mg

Hummus

Serves: As needed
Preparation time: 5 minutes
Cooking time: 0 minutes

Ingredients

1 (15-ounce) can chickpeas, drained and rinsed
⅜ cup tahini
Juice of 1 lemon
2 tablespoons cannabis olive oil
½ teaspoon ground black pepper
¼ teaspoon cayenne pepper
2 tablespoons Italian parsley, minced
1 teaspoon garlic, minced
¾ teaspoon salt
1 tablespoon extra-virgin olive oil (optional)
¼ teaspoon paprika (optional)

Directions

1. To a blender or processor, add the chickpeas, tahini, lemon juice, parsley, cannabis olive oil garlic, salt, black pepper and cayenne.
2. Blend to make a thick mixture.
3. Transfer to a mixing bowl; mix in the olive oil and top with the paprika.
4. Refrigerate for later use.

Nutrition (per tablespoon)

Calories 86
Carbs 8.6g, Fat 4.6g, Protein 3.8g, Sodium 63mg

Honey Oat Balls

Serves: As needed
Preparation time: 20 minutes
Cooking time: 5 minutes

Ingredients
1½ cups canna butter
3 cups rolled oats
2 tablespoons cocoa powder
¼ cup peanut butter
3 tablespoons honey
Cooking spray

Directions
1. Grease a baking pan with some cooking spray.
2. In a medium skillet or saucepan, melt the butter over medium heat.
3. Add the rest the ingredients, gently mix, and cook while stirring for 5 minutes.
4. Cool down completely and form into small balls.
5. Arrange on the baking pan and refrigerate for 15 minutes.
6. Serve.

Nutrition (per serving) (4 ounces)
Calories 227
Carbs 28.4g, Fat 5.6g, Protein 5.6g, Sodium 39mg

Deviled Eggs

Serves: 6
Preparation time: 15 minutes
Cooking time: 0 minutes

Ingredients
6 hard-boiled eggs
¾ teaspoon apple cider vinegar
¼ teaspoon sugar
3 tablespoons mayonnaise
¾ teaspoon Dijon mustard
Ground black pepper to taste
Pinch of decarboxylated kief or buds, crumbled
⅛ teaspoon paprika
¾ teaspoon prepared horseradish (optional)

Directions
1. Make halves from the eggs and scoop out the yolks into a mixing bowl.
2. Mix in the mayonnaise, mustard, horseradish, cider vinegar, sugar, salt, pepper and crumbled buds/kief.
3. Mash the mixture and spoon it back into the egg whites.
4. Top with the paprika and serve.

Nutrition (per serving)
Calories 88
Carbs 0.2g, Fat 8.4g, Protein 5.6g, Sodium 72mg

Sweet and Spicy Mixed Nuts

Serves: 6
Preparation time: 10 minutes
Baking time: 25 minutes

Ingredients
¼ cup packed dark brown sugar
1 tablespoon water
2 tablespoons unsalted butter
1 tablespoon cannabutter
⅛–¼ teaspoon cayenne pepper
3 cups mixed nuts (walnuts, cashew, almonds, etc.)
Salt to taste

Directions
1. Preheat oven to 300°F or 148°C. Line a large baking sheet with parchment paper.
2. In a medium skillet or saucepan, melt the cannabutter and butter over medium heat.
3. Add the brown sugar, water and cayenne.
4. Bring to a boil; cook while stirring for about 20 seconds.
5. Place the nuts in a mixing bowl and mix with the salt. Pour in the sugar sauce and coat well.
6. Arrange the coated nuts over the baking sheet in a uniform layer.
7. Bake for 8–10 minutes. Stir the nuts and bake for 15 more minutes.
8. Serve warm.

Nutrition (per serving)
Calories 376
Carbs 16.4g, Fat 28.7g, Protein 8.3g, Sodium 206mg

Baked Spinach Dip

Serves: As needed
Preparation time: 8–10 minutes
Cooking & baking time: 30–35 minutes

Ingredients

¼ teaspoon garlic, minced
4 ounces cream cheese
2 teaspoons soy sauce
1 teaspoon lemon juice
¾ cup grated parmesan cheese (divided)
¼ cup mayonnaise
1½ pounds baby spinach
Vegetable oil, as needed
2 jalapeno peppers, seeded and sliced
2 scallions, chopped
1 tablespoon cannabis coconut oil
¼ teaspoon cayenne pepper (optional)
Ground black pepper and salt to taste

Directions

1. Preheat oven to 375°F or 190°C. Grease a baking dish with some cooking spray.
2. To a medium skillet or saucepan, add the vegetable oil and heat it over medium heat.
3. Add the spinach and cook to wilt for 2 minutes. Drain additional liquid and set aside.
4. Blend the jalapenos, scallions and garlic in a food processor or blender.
5. Add the cream cheese, ½ cup of the parmesan cheese, and the cannabis coconut oil, mayonnaise, soy sauce, lemon juice, cayenne, salt and black pepper.
6. Blend to make a smooth mix.
7. Add the drained spinach and blend again.

8. Season to taste with more ground black pepper and salt.
9. Add the mixture to a baking dish and sprinkle with the remaining parmesan cheese.
10. Bake for about 25 minutes, or until bubbly.
11. Serve with your choice of crackers or bread.

Nutrition (per tablespoon)
Calories 107
Carbs 2.3g, Fat 6.4g, Protein 5.2g, Sodium 268mg

Guacamole

Serves: As needed
Preparation time: 10 minutes
Cooking time: 0 minutes

Ingredients

¼ cup red or yellow onion, finely chopped
1 small scallion, finely chopped
2 medium ripe avocados, peeled and pitted
1 medium ripe tomato, chopped
1 tablespoon cannabis coconut oil
1 tablespoon lime juice
1 medium jalapeno pepper, cored, seeded and minced
2 tablespoons chopped cilantro
¼ teaspoon minced garlic
Ground black pepper and salt to taste

Directions

1. To a food processor or blender, add the pitted avocado halves and remaining ingredients.
2. Blend or process on pulse mode until you get a firm texture. Do not over-blend.
3. Take out, season to taste, and serve.

Nutrition (per tablespoon)

Calories 42
Carbs 2.3g, Fat 3g, Protein 0.2g, Sodium 7mg

Sweet Desserts

Macadamia Choco Brownies

Serves: Makes 12 brownies
Preparation time: 8–10 minutes
Baking time: 30 minutes

Ingredients
¾ cup all-purpose flour
3 eggs
½ teaspoon vanilla extract
2 tablespoons cocoa powder
¾ teaspoon salt
⅓ cup coconut oil
¼ cup cannabis coconut oil
4½ ounces unsweetened chocolate
1 cup packed brown sugar
¾ cup chopped pecans, macadamia nuts, or almonds (optional)
Unsalted butter, melted to grease

Directions
1. Preheat oven to 350°F or 176°C. Line an 8×8 baking pan with aluminum foil and grease with some cooking spray.
2. Mix the flour, cocoa powder and salt in a mixing bowl.
3. To a medium skillet or saucepan, add both the oils and heat over medium heat.
4. Add the chocolate and cook until it melts completely.
5. Set aside to cool for 5 minutes.
6. Mix the brown sugar in with the melted chocolate.
7. Beat the eggs in a bowl and mix in the vanilla extract. Combine well.
8. Add in the flour mix and combine well; mix in the nuts.

9. Add the batter into the prepared pan and bake for 25–30 minutes, or until a toothpick comes out clean.
10. Take out and let cool; slice and serve.

Nutrition (per serving)
Calories 268
Carbs 24.6g, Fat 16.8g, Protein 3.6g, Sodium 224mg

Peanut Butter Marshmallow Lips

Serves: 6
Preparation time: 10 minutes
Cooking time: 0 minutes

Ingredients
¼ cup peanut butter
12 apple wedges
Juice of ½ lime
2 tablespoons cannabis coconut or cannabis olive oil
30 small marshmallows

Directions
1. Top the apple wedges with the lime juice.
2. In a mixing bowl, mix the peanut butter and cannabis coconut or cannabis olive oil.
3. Spread the mixture over one side of each apple wedge (not both sides).
4. Add 5 marshmallows to each spread side.
5. Place another wedge on top, with the spread side touching the marshmallows to create a lip-like appearance.
6. Repeat the same with remaining wedges.

Nutrition (per serving)
Calories 214
Carbs 34.8g, Fat 5.2g, Protein 4.1g, Sodium 66mg

Coconut Pie

Serves: Makes 1 pie (8 servings/slices)
Preparation time: 10 minutes
Cooking time: 40 minutes

Ingredients
2 cups cannabis milk
1 cup condensed milk
1 (11–12 inch) pie crust
3 large eggs
3 teaspoons vanilla extract
1 cup shredded coconut, lightly toasted
1 cup granulated sugar
½ teaspoon salt
Butter to grease

Directions
1. Preheat oven to 300°F or 148°C.
2. Grease a pie pan with some butter and place the crust in it.
3. Combine the sugar, condensed milk, cannabis milk, eggs, vanilla extract, toasted shredded coconut and salt in a mixing bowl to make a smooth mix.
4. Add the batter to the pie shell and bake for 35–40 minutes or until the pie is well set.
5. Cool down and make slices. Serve warm.

Nutrition (per serving)
Calories 523
Carbs 42.3g, Fat 26.8g, Protein 4.6g, Sodium 267mg

Classic Chocolate Chip Cookies

Serves: Makes 30 cookies
Preparation time: 10 minutes
Baking time: 12–15 minutes

Ingredients
¼ cup cannabutter, melted
¼ cup unsalted butter, melted
1 teaspoon vanilla extract
⅔ cup sugar
⅔ cup brown sugar
1 egg
½ teaspoon baking soda
½ teaspoon salt
1 cup + 2 tablespoons all-purpose flour
1 cup chocolate chips
Toasted walnuts, chopped, to taste (optional)

Directions
1. Preheat oven to 375°F or 190°C.
2. Whisk the sugar, brown sugar, canna butter, butter and vanilla extract in a mixing bowl until creamy.
3. Beat the egg in another bowl; mix with the butter mixture.
4. Stir together the flour, baking soda and salt in another bowl.
5. Mix the dry ingredients into the butter mixture to combine well.
6. Stir in the chocolate chips and nuts.
7. Drop tablespoons of dough onto 2 ungreased baking sheets; keep 1 inch between each drop.
8. Bake for 12–15 minutes until golden brown.
9. Cool on a wire rack, then serve immediately.

Nutrition (per cookie)
Calories 122
Carbs 16.3g, Fat 5.2g, Protein 1.5g, Sodium 64mg

Peach Popsicles

Serves: 6
Preparation time: 4–5 hours
Cooking time: 0 minutes

Ingredients
1 cup Greek yogurt
2 tablespoons sugar
½ cup cannabis milk
1 cup pureed peach

Directions
1. In a medium-large mixing bowl, thoroughly combine the pureed peach, cannabis milk, sugar, yogurt and vanilla extract.
2. Add the diced peaches and transfer the mixture into 6 popsicle molds.
3. Place in the freezer for 4 hours; take out and enjoy.

Nutrition (per serving)
Calories 46
Carbs 8.6g, Fat 0.3g, Protein 1g, Sodium 19mg

Red Velvet Cupcakes

Serves: 24 cupcakes
Preparation time: 10–15 minutes
Baking time: 20 minutes

Ingredients
Cupcakes
½ cup cannabis coconut or cannabis olive oil
2 eggs
1 cup buttermilk
1 cup vegetable oil
2 tablespoons red food coloring
2½ cups all-purpose flour
1½ cups sugar
⅜ cup cocoa powder
1 teaspoon distilled white vinegar
1 teaspoon vanilla extract
1 teaspoon baking soda
¾ teaspoon salt

Icing
1 teaspoon vanilla extract
8 ounces cream cheese
½ cup unsalted butter, melted
3½ cups confectioners' sugar

Directions
1. Preheat oven to 350°F or 176°C. Arrange 24 muffin cups with paper cupcake liners.
2. In a medium-large mixing bowl, thoroughly combine the buttermilk, coconut or cannabis olive oil, vegetable oil, eggs, food coloring, vinegar and vanilla extract.
3. Whisk the mixture thoroughly or use an immersion blender.

71

4. In another bowl, stir together the flour, sugar, cocoa powder, baking soda and salt. Combine the mixtures and mix just until smooth.
5. Pour the batter into the prepared muffin cups; fill them ⅔ full.
6. Bake for 20 minutes until a toothpick comes out clean.
7. Let cool completely.

Icing
1. Mix together the cream cheese, butter and vanilla extract in a mixing bowl using an electric mixer until fluffy.
2. Add the sugar and continue mixing until the sugar dissolves.
3. Spread the icing over the cupcakes and serve.

Nutrition (per serving)
Calories 323
Carbs 34.6g, Fat 16.8g, Protein 3.6g, Sodium 216mg

Coconut Chocolate Bars

Serves: 8–10
Preparation time: 15 minutes
Baking time: 30 minutes

Ingredients
1 cup chocolate chips
1 can condensed milk
1 cup graham cracker crumbs
1 cup cannabutter, melted
1 cup shredded coconut

Directions
1. Preheat oven to 350°F or 176°C.
2. Add the cannabis butter to a baking dish.
3. Add the cracker crumbs and press to form a crust.
4. Top with the coconut and chocolate chips; pour the milk over it.
5. Bake for 30 minutes or until it achieves a firm, bar-like consistency.
6. Let cool and slice into bars. Serve warm, or refrigerate and serve chilled.

Nutrition (per serving)
Calories 486
Carbs 24.6g, Fat 32.6g, Protein 3.8g, Sodium 67mg

Chocolate Fudge

Serves: 2–4
Preparation time: 10–15 minutes
Cooking time: 5 minutes

Ingredients

2–4 scoops vanilla ice cream
½ teaspoon vanilla extract
¼ cup whipped cream
¼ cup cocoa powder
Chopped nuts, to serve
½ cup corn syrup
¼ cup brown sugar
8 ounces semisweet chocolate chips
1 tablespoon cannabutter

Directions

1. To a medium skillet or saucepan, add the whipping cream, cocoa, brown sugar and corn syrup; heat over low-medium heat.
2. Let the mixture cool down.
3. Add the cannabutter, vanilla extract and chocolate; combine well to make a smooth mixture.
4. Scoop the ice cream into serving dishes; top with chocolate syrup and chopped nuts.

Nutrition (per serving)

Calories 568
Carbs 42.6g, Fat 17.6g, Protein 4.6g, Sodium 49mg

Mini Peach Cobbler

Serves: 12 mini cobblers
Preparation time: 15–20 minutes
Cooking time: 45 minutes

Ingredients
¾ cup diced peaches
1 cup all-purpose flour
1 cup + 3 tablespoons sugar
½ teaspoon cinnamon
¼ teaspoon salt
1½ teaspoons baking powder
½ teaspoon nutmeg
1 cup milk
¼ cup cannabutter, melted
¼ cup unsalted butter, melted
1 teaspoon vanilla extract
Whipped cream, to serve (optional)
Cooking spray to grease

Directions
1. Preheat oven to 350°F or 176°C. Grease 12 muffin tins with some cooking spray.
2. In a mixing bowl, mix the peaches, 3 tablespoons of sugar, and the cinnamon. Set the mixture aside.
3. In a mixing bowl, mix the flour, baking powder, 1 cup of sugar, nutmeg and salt.
4. Whisk in the milk, cannabutter, butter and vanilla extract.
5. Fill each muffin tin about half full and add the peach mixture on top.
6. Bake for 40–45 minutes until golden brown.
7. Let cool and serve.

Nutrition (per serving)
Calories 193
Carbs 24.6g, Fat 7.6g, Protein 2.7g, Sodium 63mg

Caramel Apple Dessert

Serves: 6–8
Preparation time: 10 minutes
Cooking time: 8–10 minutes

Ingredients

½ cup corn syrup
⅓ cup unsalted butter
¾ cup brown sugar
¾ cup sugar
1 tablespoon cannabutter
½ teaspoon salt
⅔ cup heavy whipping cream
4 large apples, peeled and sliced

Directions

1. To a medium skillet or saucepan, add the brown and white sugars, corn syrup, butter, cannabutter and salt and heat over medium heat.
2. Cook while stirring for 5 minutes to boil the mixture.
3. Lower heat to low and simmer for 2 more minutes.
4. Remove the pan from the heat and stir in the cream.
5. Top the apple slices with the caramel sauce; serve.

Nutrition (per serving)

Calories 453
Carbs 34.7g, Fat 14.6g, Protein 1.3g, Sodium 178mg

Recipe Index

Also by George Green

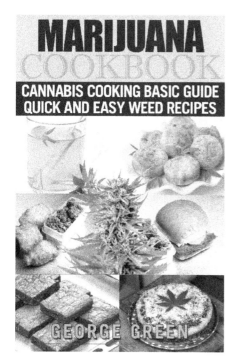

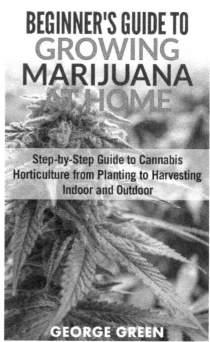

Appendix –
Cooking Conversion Charts

1. Measuring Equivalent Chart

Type	Imperial	Imperial	Metric
Weight	1 dry ounce		28 g
	1 pound	16 dry ounces	0.45 kg
Volume	1 teaspoon		5 ml
	1 dessert spoon	2 teaspoons	10 ml
	1 tablespoon	3 teaspoons	15 ml
	1 Australian tablespoon	4 teaspoons	20 ml
	1 fluid ounce	2 tablespoons	30 ml
	1 cup	16 tablespoons	240 ml
	1 cup	8 fluid ounces	240 ml
	1 pint	2 cups	470 ml
	1 quart	2 pints	0.95 l
	1 gallon	4 quarts	3.8 l
Length	1 inch		2.54 cm

* Numbers are rounded to the closest equivalent

2. Oven Temperature Equivalent Chart

Fahrenheit (°F)	Celsius (°C)	Gas Mark
220	100	
225	110	1/4
250	120	1/2
275	140	1
300	150	2
325	160	3
350	180	4
375	190	5
400	200	6
425	220	7
450	230	8
475	250	9
500	260	

* Celsius (°C) = T (°F)-32] * 5/9

** Fahrenheit (°F) = T (°C) * 9/5 + 32

*** Numbers are rounded to the closest equivalent

CPSIA information can be obtained
at www.ICGtesting.com
Printed in the USA
LVHW080103210119
604573LV00033B/619/P